STRESS RESILIENCE

Therapies for Mental Health and Well-Being

Combat Stress With A Range Of Therapeutic Strategies Designed To Promote Mental Health And Overall Well-Being

DR. BRIDGET PROMISE

Introduction

An unavoidable aspect of our daily lives in the fast-paced and demanding environment of today is stress. Stress, whether it comes from personal problems, work-related responsibilities, or unforeseen events, may negatively impact our mental health.

Nevertheless, individuals may overcome difficult circumstances and emerge stronger because of the human mind's amazing capacity for resilience. This article explores the concepts of resilience and stress, looking at how they are related and how important a part they play in determining our mental health.

Comprehending Stress And Resilience

In its most basic form, stress is the body's normal response to a perceived threat or challenge. It triggers the "fight or flight" response, a set of physiological reactions meant to prime the body to either confront or escape the stressor.

Even while this response is evolutionarily adaptable, long-term stress exposure may be detrimental to mental health.

Conversely, resilience is the ability to bounce back from adversity. It involves making positive adjustments amid hardship, tragedy, or significant life changes. Resilient people can withstand negative circumstances and bounce back, maintaining their mental health.

To develop strategies to lessen the negative impacts of stress on mental health, it is essential to comprehend the relationship between stress and resilience.

Stress's Impact On Mental Health

Stress may have detrimental effects on one's mental health, regardless of how severe or persistent it is. Long-term stress is associated with a higher chance of mental health problems, such as depression and anxiety.

High amounts of stress hormones may result from the body's stress response system being activated repeatedly. These chemicals can alter brain neurotransmitters and exacerbate mood disorders.

Moreover, stress may hinder recovery and exacerbate preexisting mental health issues. Chronic stress sufferers may find it difficult to focus, recall things, or make choices, which impairs their overall cognitive function.

Another common side effect of stress is difficulty sleeping, which exacerbates mental health concerns and may be a vicious cycle that is hard to break without professional help.

Understanding the signs of stress and how it affects mental health is essential for prompt intervention and effective therapy. There are many different ways that stress manifests itself, including irritability, mood swings, and physical symptoms like headaches and fatigue. By being aware of these signs, individuals may prevent the worsening of stress-related mental health issues by getting assistance and learning coping mechanisms.

Bases Of Resilience

Resilience protects the mental health against the damaging effects of stress. Resilience is a skill that can be cultivated and strengthened over time, even though some individuals are naturally more resilient than others. Comprehending the foundations of resilience provides individuals with a roadmap to enhance their ability to navigate life's challenges.

Resilience requires having a positive outlook on life and being mentally well. Resilience may be aided by optimism and self-belief in one's ability to overcome adversity. Building a solid support system and strong social ties is another essential stage. Reliable relationships reduce stress and provide emotional support when things are hard.

Among resilience's essential elements are flexibility and adaptability. Although life is inherently unpredictable, those who possess resilience can adapt to change while also growing from their experiences.

Building resilience may also be aided by developing a feeling of meaning and purpose in life. Being well aware of one's values and goals provides a solid base for handling challenging circumstances.

CHAPTER TWO

Psychoeducation For Mental Health And Stress Management

To empower individuals to take charge of their well-being, psychoeducation—the dissemination of information and understanding about mental health, stress, and resilience—is essential.

Psychoeducation raises consciousness and cognition, giving individuals the knowledge and abilities they need to manage stress.

To educate individuals about stress, it is necessary to look at its many internal and external origins. Internal stressors include negative thought habits, perfectionism, and personal expectations; external stressors include interpersonal roadblocks, financial difficulties, and pressure from the workplace. Identifying and categorizing these stressors enables individuals to create specialized coping mechanisms.

Psychoeducation also delves into the physiological aspects of stress, explaining how it affects the body and the psyche. A deeper comprehension of the functions of neurotransmitters, the autonomic nervous system, and stress hormones enables individuals to see the connections between mental and physical health. With this knowledge, individuals may make informed decisions about changing their lifestyles to become more resilient and less susceptible to the negative effects of stress.

Psychoeducation also emphasizes the need to get professional assistance when needed. People may find it helpful to use certain techniques and coping strategies provided by mental health professionals, whether via counseling, therapy, or other types of intervention. Normalizing the process of seeking therapy reduces stigma and encourages proactive mental health care.

In summary, stress and resilience are vital aspects of life that are closely linked to mental health. Promoting mental well-being requires accepting psychoeducation, realizing the impact of stress, and comprehending the principles of resilience. By encouraging resilience and arming people with the knowledge they need to manage stress, we can provide the foundation for better, more fulfilling lives.

Stress has become an inevitable part of life for many individuals in today's fast-paced and demanding society. Stress management is essential for overall health, and there are several ways to control and lessen the pressures that life may place on you.

This article explores the relationship between physical fitness and stress resilience, the impact of nutrition on mental health, the importance of sleep in enhancing stress resilience, and cognitive-behavioral approaches to stress management. It also covers mindfulness and meditation techniques.

Cognitive-Behavioral Stress Reduction Techniques:

Cognitive-behavioral therapy (CBT) is a well-recognized and successful method of managing stress. Cognitive Behavioral Therapy (CBT) aims to identify and address harmful thought patterns and behaviors that lead to stress.

By changing these behaviors, people may be able to better control their emotional responses and coping strategies.

CBT may assist individuals in identifying and reframing stress-inducing irrational thoughts. An example of a repetitive concept that CBT helps people address is "I must be perfect at everything I do." This belief can be replaced with a more realistic and adaptive one, such as "It's okay not to be perfect; I can learn and improve over time."

Behavioral techniques for stress reduction are also a part of CBT. These might include imparting skills in problem-solving, time management, and relaxing methods. Through the treatment of both behavioral and cognitive components, CBT provides individuals with a comprehensive toolkit for efficiently managing and reducing stress.

Practices Of Mindfulness And Meditation

The benefits of mindfulness and meditation as stress-reduction strategies have drawn a lot of attention in recent years. Conversely, meditation encompasses a range of practices intended to promote calmness of mind, relaxation, and increased consciousness.

Your ability to remain composed and resilient in the face of stress may improve with regular mindfulness and meditation practice. Mindful breathing, body scan meditations, and guided imagery are among the techniques that might assist individuals in increasing their awareness of their thoughts and feelings. This heightened consciousness facilitates a more methodical and less instinctive response to obstacles.

Research suggests that practicing mindfulness and meditation might alter brain physiology in a way that strengthens the body's ability to withstand stress. Frequent practitioners often report less anxiety, improved emotional regulation, and an overall sense of well-being. Including mindfulness in routine tasks might aid in building resilience against the negative effects of stress.

CHAPTER THREE

Physical Well-Being And Stress Management:

It is well known that resistance to stress and physical fitness are related. Frequent exercise has several benefits for mental and physical well-being. Because exercise releases endorphins, the body's natural mood boosters, it is a natural stress reliever.

Stress chemicals such as cortisol and adrenaline are also lowered by exercise. Additionally, it enhances the quality of sleep, which is crucial for stress resistance. Engaging in consistent physical activity, such as jogging or cycling, weight training, or mind-body techniques like yoga, may greatly enhance an individual's capacity to manage stress.

By concentrating attention on the body's movements and sensations, exercise itself may be used as a kind of meditation that promotes awareness. Moreover, a fitness regimen's feeling of achievement and boosted self-worth might enhance a person's general perspective on life and promote stress resistance.

The Effects Of Nutrition On Mental Health

Research on the connection between diet and mental health is expanding quickly. The health of our brains generally and the activity of neurotransmitters are greatly influenced by the food we eat. The emotional and cognitive health of an individual is enhanced by eating a diet rich in vital nutrients and well-balanced.

Certain vitamins and minerals, such as the B-complex vitamins and omega-3 fatty acids found in fish, have been linked to improved mood and stress tolerance.

Conversely, diets heavy in sugar, processed foods, and saturated fats may worsen mental health by causing inflammation.

Stress management may also be aided by eating a balanced diet that keeps blood sugar levels steady. Changes in blood sugar levels may lead to mood swings and irritation, which can intensify stress.

Eating complete, nutrient- and fiber-rich meals may help control blood sugar levels and promote emotional stability.

To put it simply, eating with awareness and purpose may be a very effective part of a comprehensive stress-reduction plan. A nutritious diet may greatly enhance mental resilience in the face of life's obstacles when paired with other lifestyle considerations.

Sleep's Beneficial Effect On Stress Resilience

A vital component of general health, sleep is also essential for stress resiliency. For emotional control, cognitive function, and general physical health, getting enough sleep is crucial. Prolonged sleep deprivation has been linked to elevated stress levels, compromised cognitive function, and an exaggerated emotional reaction to difficult circumstances.

The body goes through processes that heal and revitalize the mind and body when we sleep. This involves the processing of newly formed memories, the removal of harmful substances from the brain, and the control of stress-related hormones. Thus, obtaining enough sleep regularly is essential to developing stress tolerance.

Better sleep hygiene may be achieved by developing a regular sleep schedule, making your bedroom cozy, and using relaxation methods before bed. A more peaceful night's sleep may be achieved by limiting screen time before bed, abstaining from stimulants like coffee in the evening, and reducing stress with relaxation or mindfulness practices.

In summary, a mix of cognitive-behavioral techniques, mindfulness and meditation exercises, regular exercise, a healthy diet, and placing a high priority on getting enough sleep are all part of the holistic approach to stress management.

People may develop a stronger feeling of inner balance and

serenity, improve their general quality of life, and become more resilient to stress by addressing many facets of life and well-being.

CHAPTER FOUR

Creating Healthy Connections To Provide Emotional Support

It is impossible to overestimate the significance of good connections in life's journey. A vital component of emotional health is human connection, which is essential for giving one the support one needs to deal with the challenges of day-to-day living.

Building a network of supporting people is crucial for emotional resilience, both in personal and professional interactions. We explore many aspects of creating and sustaining good relationships in this investigation, highlighting the variety of support systems that enhance emotional wellness.

Professional Assistance: Counseling And Therapy

Getting professional assistance when necessary is a fundamental component of creating strong connections for emotional support.

Counseling and therapy provide people with controlled, private spaces to examine their feelings, ideas, and experiences. Professional therapists provide a safe, nonjudgmental environment while providing strategies and resources for handling difficulties, stress reduction, and improving emotional toughness.

Different types of therapy are available to meet the requirements and preferences of individuals. The goal of cognitive-behavioral therapy, or CBT, is to recognize and alter harmful thinking processes and behavior patterns.

By examining how previous experiences shape current behavior, psychodynamic therapy promotes self-awareness and understanding. In addition, there are specialty types of treatment including group, family, and couples therapy, each of which is intended to address a particular relationship dynamic.

Counseling offers a safe space for talking about issues, getting perspective, and creating coping mechanisms, whether it is individual or group-focused. Individuals are encouraged to actively participate in their personal development and problem-solving processes through the collaborative character of counseling. Seeking expert assistance is a proactive move toward preserving general well-being and developing emotional resilience rather than a show of weakness.

Holistic Methods For Developing Stress Resilience

Holistic methods, in addition to expert assistance, are essential for promoting mental well-being. Taking into account how the mind, body, and spirit are interrelated is essential to holistic well-being. Developing habits that take care of these interrelated areas builds resistance to stress and a feeling of equilibrium in one's life.

One such all-encompassing strategy is mindfulness

meditation, which is widely known for its advantages in lowering stress and fostering emotional health. Through growing awareness without passing judgment, this technique invites people to be present in the moment. Frequent mindfulness meditation has been associated with enhanced self-awareness, calmer feelings, and better emotional control.

An additional essential element of holistic well-being is physical exercise. Exercise has been shown to produce endorphins, which are the body's natural mood enhancers and may lower stress and foster a cheerful perspective. Particularly yoga and tai chi integrate physical exercise with mindfulness, which has positive effects on the body as well as the mind.

The Mind-Body Link: Tai Chi And Yoga

Ancient techniques like yoga and tai chi highlight the mind-body link and provide a comprehensive approach to mental and physical health. Through deliberate movement, deliberate breathing, and mindfulness, these activities help people develop a feeling of harmony and balance within themselves.

Yoga is an ancient Indian philosophy that consists of breathing techniques, postures, and meditation. The focus on breathwork improves awareness and relaxation, while the physical postures, or asanas, encourage flexibility and strength. Yoga is an effective technique for lowering stress and anxiety levels and fostering emotional resilience because it combines meditation with physical exercise.

Chinese martial techniques are the source of tai chi, which is characterized by slow, flowing motions and deep breathing. Tai Chi, also called "meditation in motion," enhances mental clarity, flexibility, and balance. Because of its soothing and rhythmic style, Tai Chi is suitable for people of all ages and fitness levels and provides a very beneficial, low-impact method of improving the mind-body connection.

Adding yoga or Tai Chi to your regimen is a great way to take care of your mental health in addition to your physical health.

CHAPTER FIVE

Creative Expression And Art Therapy

Within the field of emotional support, art therapy offers a distinctive and potent means of facilitating self-exploration and healing via artistic expression. Using a variety of artistic mediums, including painting, sketching, sculpture, and even music, art therapy enables people to explore and express their feelings nonverbally.

Expressing oneself creatively gives emotions an outlet that could be difficult to communicate verbally.

Instead of emphasizing the production of masterpieces, art therapy concentrates on the creative process and the feelings that surface when exploring one's artistic side. By encouraging people to use their natural creativity, this type of therapy helps people better understand their feelings and gives them a sense of success.

Art therapy works especially well for those who may have trouble vocally expressing their emotions. The process of making art enables the symbolic portrayal of feelings, giving therapists important insights into the client's inner world. The material results of the creative process can act as a visible reminder of perseverance and personal development.

In summary, developing wholesome connections for emotional support requires a diversified strategy that incorporates holistic methods, professional assistance, and artistic expression. While holistic practices like yoga and Tai Chi promote the mind-body connection necessary for emotional resilience, therapy, and counseling provide organized opportunities for self-exploration and development. Through creative expression, art therapy offers a special and priceless way to comprehend and process emotions. When combined, these many approaches strengthen the foundation of a strong support network, fostering mental health and improving the general quality of life.

Nature Therapy: The Restorative Potential Of Nature

People are turning more and more to nature therapy—a discipline based on the conviction that the natural world has unmatched therapeutic abilities for the mind, body, and spirit—for comfort in the fast-paced, contemporary world where stress and worry appear to be permanent companions. The idea is not new; ancient societies have long understood the healing powers of spending time outside.

These days, people are grappling with the pressures of a technologically-driven lifestyle and rising stress levels, which is why nature therapy is becoming more important.

Spirituality And Resilience To Stress

The powerful effects of nature therapy on stress resilience and spirituality are one important factor to consider. People who interact with nature often experience awe and amazement, which strengthens their feeling of connection to something bigger than themselves.

A sensation of transcendence or unity with the cosmos might be a part of this spiritual connection. Studies indicate that those who integrate nature into their spiritual practices have higher levels of stress resilience and are better equipped to handle life's obstacles.

The peacefulness of natural environments promotes awareness and helps people to remain in the present moment. Whether it's a tranquil forest, a bubbling creek, or an amazing mountain view, these natural settings have the power to inspire serenity and help people unplug from the strains of everyday life.

By doing this, individuals often find that they have a fresh perspective on life and are better equipped to handle its challenges with grace and resiliency.

Tools & Technology For Stress Reduction

Going back to nature for stress relief may seem strange in a world where technology rules. Nevertheless, incorporating tools and technology into nature therapy has emerged as a potent and practical way to increase its efficacy.

Applications for smartphones that provide guided nature excursions, mindfulness exercises, and meditation have grown in popularity. These applications use technology to help people interact with nature, even while they're in city settings. As a method for reducing stress, virtual reality experiences that mimic natural environments have also gained popularity. These experiences enable people to lose themselves in the sights and sounds of nature without ever leaving their homes.

When necessary, wearable technology with biometric sensors can monitor physiological reactions to stress and motivate users to partake in outdoor activities. With the real-time input these technologies provide, people may become more aware of their stress levels and take proactive steps toward self-care.

The need for balance is becoming more apparent despite the widespread use of technology. Virtual experiences may be beneficial, but they might not be able to completely replace the tactile, multisensory engagement that comes from being in the real world. Achieving comprehensive stress management requires finding a balance between the genuineness of the natural world and the convenience of technology.

CHAPTER SIX

Developing A Mentality Of Resilience

Beyond only offering brief stress relief, nature therapy encourages the development of a resilient attitude that can face obstacles in life.

Frequent exposure to natural environments has been associated with higher problem-solving abilities, increased creativity, and improved cognitive function. These cognitive advantages support a person's general mental resilience, allowing them to tackle challenges with flexibility and clarity.

Important lessons about impermanence and the cyclical nature of life may be learned from the rhythmic rhythms of nature, such as the tide's ebb and flow and the seasons' changes.

Acceptance and adaptability are essential elements of a resilient mentality, and they may be cultivated by embracing these natural patterns. People may be motivated to overcome their challenges with bravery and tenacity by seeing the natural world's resiliency.

Furthermore, physical activities in natural environments, like hiking, gardening, or just taking a leisurely walk, encourage the production of endorphins, which are endogenous hormones that are known to elevate mood.

Engaging in physical exercise and spending time outside may create a positive feedback loop that strengthens a resilient mentality, enabling people to manage stress more effectively.

In Summary

The idea of nature therapy provides a novel and useful method of stress management in a society where stress has almost become a given. Beyond its physical effects, the outdoors has a therapeutic force that affects spirituality, stress resilience, and mental health in general.

With more people realizing the value of preserving a connection with the natural world, nature therapy is using technology and resources in creative ways to make these experiences available to a wider range of people.

The holistic approach to health that nature therapy promotes emphasizes the connection between the mind, body, and spirit. Through consistent exposure to natural surroundings, people may develop a resilient attitude that equips them with the mental toughness necessary to overcome obstacles in life.

One thing is certain as we delve more into the complex interactions between technology, nature, and stress reduction: the outdoors' healing potential is an ageless and priceless tool for building robust, well-balanced lives.